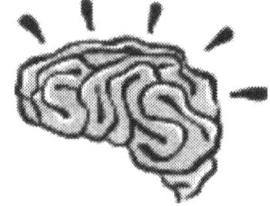

BrainReady

BrainChallenge

Helping you fight mental aging - the easy
& convenient way

Jim Balabuszko-Reay
and Paul Sebastien

Written by Jim Balabuszko-Reay
and Paul Sebastien

www.brainready.com
info@brainready.com

Published by Lulu.com
www.lulu.com

ISBN: 978-1-4303-1413-4

Welcome!
Ready for a Challenge?

The brain is a wonderful thing. Just think where you'd be without one! But starting from around age 25, our brains begin to deteriorate, with each passing year: memory, speed, recall, overall brainpower. Fortunately, recent research has shown that there's actually something you can do about that: brain exercises!

Exercise is not just for bodies anymore. Studies have shown that doing creative, spatial and memory-challenging exercises can actually help prevent brain deterioration and even help recover lost function. That's right: just like your physical body, it's "Use it or Lose it".

Interestingly, studies have also shown that traditional brain teasers and tough puzzles are not as beneficial to brain health as repeated, simpler exercises that work *several* areas of the brain. Just like doing a comprehensive physical cross-training workout is better for your overall health than, say, only doing bench presses.

With this in mind, we have created these BrainChallenge exercises, intended to help you cross train your brain while making it FUN, and easy. You won't find any trivia here, nor any math, logic, or any other puzzles. This book is dedicated to exercising your memory and creativity. The only think you'll need is a pencil and your brain.

Here's what you'll find in the pages that follow...

Recall:

In these exercises, you're challenged to recall events from long ago or earlier today, from major life events to everyday details. Variations include answering short questions, writing out longer stories, or drawing objects from memory.

The ultimate goal is not just to remember these items, but to *unclog and reawaken* your memory capacity, which can help your past, present and future memory power!

Creative

Drawing, creative writing, poetry – it's all here to help exercise your brain. Don't worry if you don't feel like an "artist" - the important thing is that you just *try* each one. These challenges deliver a truly comprehensive workout for your brain.

Switch-Up

Some exercises ask that you do it twice: from writing from two points of view, drawing multiple sides of an object, to drawing and writing with both hands. These force you to use different areas of your brain and really fire those synapses in new ways!

Spatial

These exercises force your brain to consider your environment, past & present, and draw maps – recalling a sense of space, how disparate elements relate to one another in the abstract and practical, really pushing your spatial abilities forward!

We hope you enjoy these exercises, and that doing them helps you truly FEEL your brain re-awakening. But most importantly, we hope that you HAVE FUN cross-training your brain!

For more information on Brain Health, be sure to visit
www.brainready.com

Now, on to the BrainChallenge!

Category: Recall   **Difficulty: Medium**

Draw your key ring and all keys on it.

Drawing from Memory exercises your critical Spatial and Memory brain areas as well as brain-motor skills. This one is a true cross-brain workout! Just try your best.

What were you doing today at 7:30am?

_____

_____

_____

_____

What were you doing at noon yesterday?

_____

_____

_____

_____

It can be surprising how short-term details can be *harder* to recall than older, but larger, life events. Spend a few moments and really try to remember the details...

BrainChallenge™ - Life Map

Category: Spatial   **Difficulty: Easy**

Draw a Map: From your home
to your favorite restaurant

Be as detailed as you can - imagine yourself traveling this
route! See it in your mind's eye...

BrainChallenge™ - Haiku

Category: Creative	Difficulty: Easy

Write a Haiku about Summer

_____

_____

_____

Now, write a Haiku about the Sun

_____

_____

_____

HOW TO HAIKU:

Haiku is a Japanese Poetry Form:
The first line is 5 syllables
The second line is 7 syllables
The third is 5
It need not rhyme!

Writing in haiku forces you to think differently about language, to express yourself in a new way, which is an *excellent* creative, translative exercise for your brain!

Category: Recall   Difficulty: Medium

Who was your first schoolyard crush?

_____

What color was his/her hair?

_____

What color were his/her eyes?

_____

What year was this?

_____

Don't worry if you can't recall every detail right away. You may find that as you do other unrelated exercises, these memories will come to you. That's your brain unclogging those cobwebs!

Category: Switch-Up   **Difficulty: Medium**

Draw a FACE with your LEFT HAND

Drawing the same object with the right and left hand illustrates
how hand preference is "hard wired" into our brains....

Category: Switch-Up   **Difficulty: Medium**

Draw a FACE with your RIGHT HAND

... and by forcing your non-dominant hand to try to do the same task as your dominant one, you are forcing your brain into a tough, comprehensive "adaptation" workout!

What did you do for your 16th Birthday?

_____

_____

_____

_____

_____

_____

_____

_____

_____

_____

Don't worry if you can't recall every detail right away. You may find that as you do other unrelated exercises, these answers may come to you...

Write 7 Adjectives that describe Your Best Friend.

_____

_____

_____

_____

_____

_____

_____

Coming up with alternate ways to describe important things in our lives can be hard work. Feel free to write more than seven, if you can!

Category: Recall **Difficulty: Hard**

Write in as many languages as you can:
Hello!

_____

_____

_____

_____

_____

_____

_____

_____

_____

Learning and using languages is great brain exercise.

If you don't know any other languages, why not think of several ways to say it in your own language?

Category: Recall   Difficulty: Medium

Draw the label of the most recent bottled beverage you enjoyed.

Drawing from Memory exercises hand-eye coordination, and pushes you to recall fine detail as well as general size and shape relationships. No peeking at the bottle!

Category: Switch-Up   Difficulty: Medium

Why are Cars better than Bicycles?

_____

_____

_____

_____

_____

_____

_____

_____

_____

_____

In point counterpoint, try to make a good case for BOTH SIDES
of the argument. It forces you to examine your assumptions
and bias...

Why are Bicycles better than Cars?

_____

_____

_____

_____

_____

_____

_____

_____

_____

_____

By giving a small area to write, your brain is forced to channel creativity and information prioritization!

BrainChallenge™ - Life Map

Category: Spatial   Difficulty: Medium

Draw a Map: From your home to work

(If you're not working, how about school, church, or a community center?)

Be as detailed as you can - but no need to keep to scale, since this isn't a very big box...

What did you have for dinner two nights ago?

_____

_____

_____

_____

How about four nights ago?

_____

_____

_____

_____

It can be surprising how short term details can be harder to recall than larger life events. Spend a few moments and really try to remember these details.

Category: Switch-Up   **Difficulty: Easy**

1	2	3
4	5	6
7	8	9

Write out the numbers 1-9

Writing with the right and left hand shows some unique ways in which hand preference is "hard wired" into our brains....

Category: Switch-Up   **Difficulty: Easy**

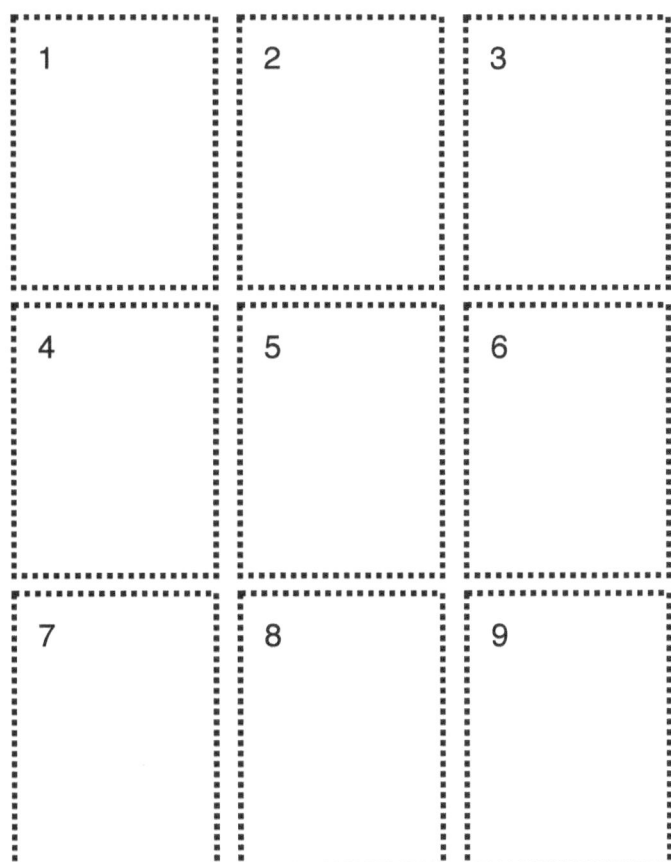

Write out the numbers 1-9

Interesting how something we see and write every day like
numbers can be so difficult to do with your non-dominant hand,
isn't it?

Category: Creative   **Difficulty: Medium**

Write exactly 25 words about:
Your Favorite Color

_____

_____

_____

_____

_____

_____

_____

_____

_____

_____

Expressing yourself within a fixed set of rules can force you to explore different words and sentence structures, which is good brain exercise.

Category: Creative	Difficulty: Medium

Write a Haiku about anything...
and use the word "Powerful"

_____

_____

_____

Now, write a Haiku about electricity:

_____

_____

_____

HOW TO:

Haiku is a Japanese Poetry Form:
The first line is 5 syllables
The second line is 7 syllables
The third is 5
It need not rhyme!

Writing in verse or haiku forces you to think differently about language, to express yourself in a new way, which is excellent exercise for your brain!

Category: Creative   **Difficulty: Easy**

Draw a Mouse

Drawing from Memory exercises hand-eye coordination, and pushes you to recall fine detail as well as general size and shape relationships. Just try your best!.

BrainChallenge™ - Milestones

Category: Recall   **Difficulty: Medium**

What was your first job outside the home?

_____

Who was your employer?

_____

What were you paid?

_____

What year was this?

_____

Don't worry if you can't bring to mind every detail right away.
You may find that as you do other unrelated exercises, these
answers come to you. That's your brain getting more fit!

Category: Switch-Up   Difficulty: Medium

Draw a Coin from Memory

Drawing from Memory exercises hand-eye coordination, and
pushes you to recall fine detail.

Category: Switch-Up   Difficulty: Medium

Draw the FLIP SIDE of that coin

We tend to memorize just key details about common objects.
Visualizing objects from multiple angles can be a good mental
challenge.

Write 7 Adjectives that describe Your Feet.

_____

_____

_____

_____

_____

_____

_____

Coming up with alternate ways to describe important (or mundane) things in our lives can be hard work.

Category: Recall   Difficulty: Hard

What did you do for your most recent Birthday?

_____

_____

_____

_____

_____

_____

_____

_____

_____

Feel free to come back to this later if the details are fuzzy... As you do other exercises, your memory will be sparked!

Category: Spatial   **Difficulty: Hard**

Draw a Map: From your Childhood home to one parent's workplace

Be as detailed as you can...

Write exactly 25 words about:
Your Favorite Musician

_____

_____

_____

_____

_____

_____

_____

_____

_____

Expressing yourself within a fixed set of rules can force you to explore different words and sentence structures, which is good brain exercise.

Category: Switch-Up	Difficulty: Medium

Why are Dogs better than Cats?

_____

_____

_____

_____

_____

_____

_____

_____

_____

_____

In point counterpoint, try to make a good case for BOTH SIDES
of the argument. It forces you to examine your assumptions
and bias...

Why are Cats better than Dogs?

_____

_____

_____

_____

_____

_____

_____

_____

_____

_____

By giving a small area to write, we are encouraging economy
in writing and creative wording.

Category: Recall   Difficulty: Hard

Write in as many languages as you can:
Goodbye!

_____

_____

_____

_____

_____

_____

_____

_____

_____

Learning and using languages is great brain exercise.

If you don't know any other languages, why not think of as many ways to say it in your own language?

What were the most recent words you said to another person today?

_____

_____

_____

_____

What time did you first speak to another person today, and what was the situation?

_____

_____

_____

_____

Spend a few moments and really try to remember these details.

BrainChallenge™ - Left Hand Drawing

Category: Switch-Up   Difficulty: Medium

Draw a TREE with your LEFT HAND

Drawing the same object with the right and left hand shows
some unique ways in which hand preference is "hard wired"
into our brains....

Category: Switch-Up   Difficulty: Medium

Draw a TREE with your RIGHT HAND

... and by forcing your non-dominant hand to try to do the
same task as your dominant one, you are actually working
some seldom used areas of your brain

Category: Creative   Difficulty: Easy

Write a Haiku about Ice

_____

_____

_____

Now, write a Haiku about Glass

_____

_____

_____

HOW TO HAIKU:

Haiku is a Japanese Poetry Form:
The first line is 5 syllables
The second line is 7 syllables
The third is 5
It need not rhyme!

Writing in verse or haiku forces you to think differently about language, to express yourself in a new way, which is excellent exercise for your brain!

Category: Recall   Difficulty: Medium

Draw the manufacturer's logo of the last automobile you owned.

Drawing from Memory exercises hand-eye coordination, and pushes you to recall fine detail as well as general size and shape relationships.

Category: Recall   Difficulty: Medium

What was your first Research Paper about?

_____

What grade did you write it in?

_____

What grade did you receive?

_____

What was your teacher's name?

_____

You may find that as you do other exercises, these answers
come to you. That's your brain getting more fit!

BrainChallenge™ - Seven Adjectives

Category: Creative   **Difficulty: Easy**

Write 7 Adjectives that describe
Your Last Night's Sleep.

_____

_____

_____

_____

_____

_____

Coming up with alternate ways to describe important things in
our lives can be hard work. Feel free to write more!

Category: Recall   Difficulty: Medium

Draw the Eiffel Tower

Try to remember key details - how many levels, how the girders and arches are formed...

Category: Creative   Difficulty: Hard

Write 25 words about Your Next Adventure

_____

_____

_____

_____

_____

_____

_____

_____

_____

_____

Let your imagination run wild... within 25 words of course!
Working creatively within constraints is a great workout.

BrainChallenge™ - Left Hand Writing

Category: Switch Up   **Difficulty: Medium**

Write with your LEFT Hand:

The Title of your Favorite Song, along with the Artist, and Album

_____

_____

_____

Writing with the right and left hand shows some unique ways in which hand preference is "hard wired" into our brains....

Category: Switch Up   **Difficulty:** Medium

Write with your RIGHT Hand:

The Title of your Favorite Song, along with the Artist, and Album

_____

_____

_____

It's amazing how the same words and letters can look so different when produced by your non-dominant hand, isn't it?

BrainChallenge™ - Life Map Recall

Category: Spatial   **Difficulty: Medium**

Draw a Map: From your home to your best friend's house when you were 14

A double challenge: Remembering your life from back then AND recalling spacial details.

BrainChallenge™ - Language

Category: Recall   **Difficulty: Hard**

Write in as many languages as you can:
I Love You

_____

_____

_____

_____

_____

_____

_____

_____

_____

_____

Learning and using languages is great brain exercise.

If you don't know any other languages, why not think of as many ways to say it in your own language?

Category: Switch-Up   **Difficulty:** Medium

Why is Red better than Blue?

_____

_____

_____

_____

_____

_____

_____

_____

_____

Try to make a good case for BOTH SIDES of the argument. It
forces you to examine your assumptions and bias...

Why is Blue better than Red?

_____

_____

_____

_____

_____

_____

_____

_____

_____

_____

This time, it's a completely non-controversial topic, and you'll
be challenged to make a case for either side... but still you
must try!

BrainChallenge™ - Haiku

Category: Creative   **Difficulty: Easy**

Write a Haiku about Sadness

_____

_____

_____

Now, write a Haiku using the following two words: "Tears" "Rain"

_____

_____

_____

HOW TO HAIKU:

Haiku is a Japanese Poetry Form:
The first line is 5 syllables
The second line is 7 syllables
The third is 5

Writing in verse or haiku forces you to think differently about language, to express yourself in a new way, which is excellent exercise for your brain!

What was the very last image you saw on television before turning it off?

_____

_____

_____

What was the very last thing you heard on the radio before turning it off?

_____

_____

_____

Try to remember the exact last thing you saw or heard -
perhaps an advertisement, or the end-credits to a show?

Category: Recall   Difficulty: Hard

Draw the Flags of your Nation AND your State/Province

While your national flag may be easy, chances are you've never really considered your regional flag in depth. Now is the time!

Category: Creative   Difficulty: Easy

Write 7 Adjectives that describe
The View Outside Your Window.

_____

_____

_____

_____

_____

_____

_____

If you are not near a window, simply look around you.

Taking the time to notice and describe our environment is
exercise for your brain.

Category: Switch-Up   **Difficulty:** Medium

Draw a CAR with your LEFT HAND

Drawing the same object with the right and left hand shows
some unique ways in which hand preference is "hard wired"
into our brains....

Category: Switch-Up   Difficulty: Medium

Draw a CAR with your RIGHT HAND

... and by forcing your non-dominant hand to try to do the
same task as your dominant one, you are actually working
some seldom used areas of your brain

BrainChallenge™ - Twenty Five Words

Category: Creative   **Difficulty: Medium**

Write 25 words about Your Nemesis

_____

_____

_____

_____

_____

_____

_____

_____

_____

_____

If you don't have an arch-enemy, by all means invent one for
this exercise. Have fun!

Category: Recall   Difficulty: Medium

What was your last blood pressure reading?

_____

What is your blood type?

_____

What was your last cholesterol reading?

_____

What is your current weight?

_____

Your brain does inhabit your body, so you should have your
vital statistics at hand. You never know when this information
may come in useful.

Category: Recall   Difficulty: Hard

What did you do to celebrate your most recent "Decade" Birthday?

_____

_____

_____

_____

_____

_____

_____

_____

_____

_____

Remembering details about major events in your life like a decade birthday (30,40,50,60) can be surprisingly difficult! Take your time and enjoy the memory.

Category: Recall   Difficulty: Medium

Draw your home computer, and everything that's attached to it.

Drawing from Memory pushes you to recall fine detail as well as general size and shape relationships. Just try your best!.

BrainChallenge™- Haiku

Category: Creative	Difficulty: Medium

Write a Haiku about Usefulness

_____

_____

_____

Now, write a Haiku about using the words "Hands" and "Thought"

_____

_____

_____

HOW TO HAIKU:

Haiku is a Japanese Poetry Form:
The first line is 5 syllables
The second line is 7 syllables
The third is 5

Writing in verse or haiku forces you to think differently about language, to express yourself in a new way, which is excellent exercise for your brain!

Category: Spatial   **Difficulty: Medium**

Draw a Map: From your home to your favorite grocery store.

Be as detailed as you can - put in landmarks as you can..

BrainChallenge™ - Left Hand Writing

| Category: Switch Up | Difficulty: Hard |

Sign your NAME with your LEFT Hand:
Four times please:

_____

_____

_____

_____

Writing with the right and left hand shows some unique ways in which hand preference is "hard wired" into our brains, and your signature is one of the hardest to switch hands on.

Category: Switch Up   Difficulty: Hard

Sign your NAME with your RIGHT Hand:
Four times please:

_____

_____

_____

_____

It's amazing how something as common as your signature (or autograph) looks quite different when produced by your non-dominant hand.

Category: Creative   **Difficulty: Easy**

Draw an Octopus

They're not all hard: Have some fun drawing this.

Category: Creative   **Difficulty: Easy**

Write 7 Adjectives that describe Your Mood Right Now

_____

_____

_____

_____

_____

_____

_____

We take our moods for granted, and usually only have one or
two adjectives for a current state. Think hard and come up
with seven!

BrainChallenge™ - Short Term Memory

Category: Recall   **Difficulty: Easy**

Describe one piece of news you learned about today.

_____

_____

_____

_____

How did you learn about it?

_____

_____

_____

_____

Short term details can be harder to recall than larger life events. Spend a few moments and really try to remember.

Category: Creative   Difficulty: Medium

Write 25 words about Your Current Goal

_____

_____

_____

_____

_____

_____

_____

_____

_____

_____

_____

Working creatively within constraints is excellent brain exercise.
Having goals in life is excellent all-around.

Category: Switch-Up   Difficulty: Medium

Draw a piece of Currency from Memory

Drawing from Memory exercises hand-eye coordination, and
pushes you to recall fine detail.

BrainChallenge™ - Drawing Tails

Category: Switch-Up	Difficulty: Medium

Draw the OTHER SIDE of that bill

We tend to memorize just key details about common objects. Visualizing objects from multiple angles can be a good mental challenge.

BrainChallenge™ - Language

Category: Recall   Difficulty: Hard

Write in as many languages as you can:
Help!

_____

_____

_____

_____

_____

_____

_____

_____

_____

Learning and using languages is great brain exercise.

If you don't know any other languages, why not think of as many ways to say it in your own language?

Category: Creative   Difficulty: Easy

Write a Haiku about the Sky

_____

_____

_____

Now, write a Haiku about Jumping

_____

_____

_____

HOW TO HAIKU:

Haiku is a Japanese Poetry Form:
The first line is 5 syllables
The second line is 7 syllables
The third is 5
It need not rhyme!

Writing in verse or haiku forces you to think differently about language, which is excellent exercise for your brain!

Why is Guitar better than Piano?

_____

_____

_____

_____

_____

_____

_____

_____

_____

Try to make a good case for BOTH SIDES of the argument. It
forces you to examine your assumptions and bias...

Category: Switch-Up   **Difficulty: Medium**

Why is Piano better than Guitar?

_____

_____

_____

_____

_____

_____

_____

_____

_____

_____

In this case, think of musical examples, people who play both, sound, and aesthetics.

Category: Recall   Difficulty: Medium

Draw the label of your favorite soup can

Drawing from Memory pushes you to recall fine detail on common objects you may not be paying close attention to. No fair looking at the can!

Who was your first real boy/girlfriend?

_____

How did you meet?

_____

_____

_____

_____

What year was this?

_____

Don't worry if you can't recall every detail right away. You may find that as you do other unrelated exercises, these memories will come to you. That's your brain unclogging those cobwebs!

Write with your LEFT Hand:

The Title of your Favorite Movie, along with the Star, and Director

_____

_____

_____

Writing with the right and left hand shows some unique ways in which hand preference is "hard wired" into our brains....

Write with your RIGHT Hand:

The Title of your Favorite Movie,
along with the Star, and Director

_____

_____

_____

It's amazing how the same words and letters can look so
different when produced by your non-dominant hand, isn't it?

Write 7 Adjectives that describe
Your Favorite Chair

_____

_____

_____

_____

_____

_____

It can be difficult to describe the commonplace in our lives.
Take the time to really describe this object. It'll be a great
brain workout!

Category: Creative　　　　Difficulty: Easy

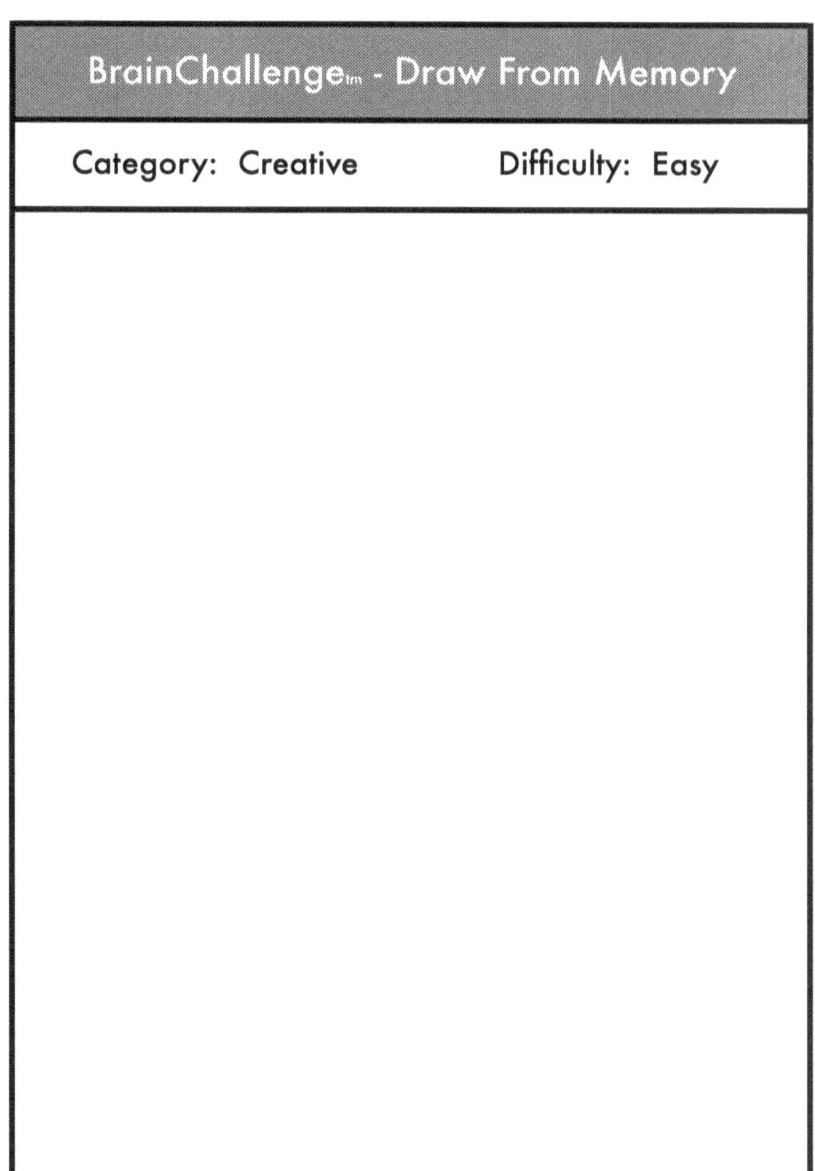

Draw a Flower

Drawing from Memory exercises hand-eye coordination, and pushes you to recall fine detail as well as general size and shape relationships.

Category: Creative　　　**Difficulty: Medium**

Write exactly 25 words about:
Your Favorite Writer

_____

_____

_____

_____

_____

_____

_____

_____

_____

Expressing yourself within a fixed set of rules can force you to explore different words and sentence structures, which is good brain exercise.

Category: Spatial   **Difficulty: Hard**

Draw a Map: From your home (at the time) to your very first Job

Be as detailed as you can - you need to recall a lot of details here - where you lived, where you worked, and how to get there!

BrainChallenge™ - Short Term Memory

Category: Recall   Difficulty: Easy

What did you eat for Breakfast today?

_____

_____

_____

_____

What did you eat for Lunch yesterday?

_____

_____

_____

_____

It can be surprising how short term details can be harder to recall than larger life events. Spend a few moments and really try to remember these details.

Category: Creative   Difficulty: Easy

Write a Haiku about Creativity

_____

_____

_____

Now, write a Haiku about Pencils

_____

_____

_____

HOW TO HAIKU:

Haiku is a Japanese Poetry Form:
The first line is 5 syllables
The second line is 7 syllables
The third is 5
It need not rhyme!

Writing in verse or haiku forces you to think differently about language, to express yourself in a new way, which is excellent exercise for your brain!

Category: Switch-Up   **Difficulty: Medium**

Draw a CAT with your LEFT HAND

Drawing the same object with the right and left hand shows some unique ways in which hand preference is "hard wired" into our brains....

Category: Switch-Up   **Difficulty: Medium**

Draw a CAT with your RIGHT HAND

... and by forcing your non-dominant hand to try to do the same task as your dominant one, you are actually working some seldom used areas of your brain.

What did you do for your 21st Birthday?

_____

_____

_____

_____

_____

_____

_____

_____

_____

_____

Don't worry if you can't recall every detail right away. It must
have been a great party. Let the details come to you naturally.

Category: Recall   **Difficulty: Hard**

Write in as many languages as you can:
Yes and No

_____

_____

_____

_____

_____

_____

_____

_____

_____

Learning and using languages is great brain exercise.

If you don't know any other languages, why not think of as
many ways to say it in your own language?

Category: Recall   Difficulty: Medium

Draw the Taj Mahal

Drawing from Memory pushes you to recall fine detail on
familiar objects. How many domes?

Write exactly 25 words about:
Your Best Laugh

_____

_____

_____

_____

_____

_____

_____

_____

_____

_____

Expressing yourself within a fixed set of rules can force you to explore different words and sentence structures, which is good brain exercise.

Why were the '60s better than the '70s?

_____

_____

_____

_____

_____

_____

_____

_____

_____

_____

Try to make a good case for BOTH SIDES of the argument. It
forces you to examine your assumptions and bias...

Why were the '70s better than the '60s?

_____

_____

_____

_____

_____

_____

_____

_____

_____

_____

In this case, you may need to overcome strong bias to make one point over the other. The more you stretch yourself, the better the exercise for your brain!.

Category: Spatial   **Difficulty: Hard**

Draw a Map: From your home (at the time) to school when you were 12 years old.

Be as detailed as you can - but no need to keep to scale, since this isn't a very big box...

Who was the last person you spoke with on the phone?

_____

Who initiated the call?

_____

Did you laugh during the call?

_____

How did you sign off the call?

_____

Sometimes the more everyday details of our lives are the hardest to remember. Give it a try!

Category: Recall   Difficulty: Easy

Draw your bedside lamp

Drawing from Memory exercises hand-eye coordination, and pushes you to recall fine detail as well as general size and shape relationships. Just try your best!.

Category: Creative   **Difficulty: Easy**

Write a Haiku about the Night Sky

_____

_____

_____

Now, write a Haiku about using the words "Saturn" and "Earth"

_____

_____

_____

HOW TO HAIKU:

Haiku is a Japanese Poetry Form:
The first line is 5 syllables
The second line is 7 syllables
The third is 5

Writing in verse or haiku forces you to think differently about language, to express yourself in a new way, which is excellent exercise for your brain!

Category: Recall   Difficulty: Hard

Write exactly 25 words about:
Your Hero

_____

_____

_____

_____

_____

_____

_____

_____

_____

Working creatively within constraints is a great workout.

Category: Recall   **Difficulty: Hard**

Write in as many languages as you can:
My Name Is...

_____

_____

_____

_____

_____

_____

_____

_____

_____

_____

Learning and using languages is great brain exercise.

If you don't know any other languages, why not think of as
many ways to say it in your own language?

Where was your first "big" job interview?

_____

Who did you interview with?

_____

What came of that interview?

_____

What did you wear?

_____

You may not be able to recall every detail right away. You may find that as you do other unrelated exercises, these answers come to you. That's your brain getting more fit!

Category: Creative   Difficulty: Medium

Draw a Spaceship

Just for fun - any kind. From a movie, or from your
imagination. Creative exercises are great brain training!

BrainChallenge™ - Seven Adjectives

Category: Creative	Difficulty: Easy

Write 7 Adjectives that describe You.

_____

_____

_____

_____

_____

_____

_____

Coming up with alternate ways to describe yourself can be hard, but you're up to the challenge!

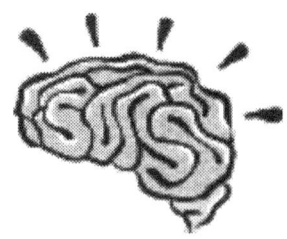

Congratulations!
You've completed the
BrainReady
BrainChallenge

Learn the latest brain health & anti-aging
nutritional advice, brain exercises, audio
brain training and much more...FREE at:
www.brainready.com

or send us an email at
info@brainready.com

Thank You!
Jim and Paul

Also Available from BrainReady.com
(printed or download versions):

BrainFlex Worksheets Volume 1
28 daily brain training worksheets

BrainChallenge 2
More creative and recall challenges to strengthen mental acuity the fun and easy way.

www.ingramcontent.com/pod-product-compliance
Lightning Source LLC
Chambersburg PA
CBHW031245280526
45784CB00004B/1730